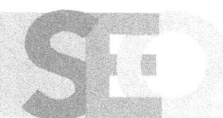

Career Health Inventory
and Development Guide (CHI)

smart 2 SMARTER
Resource Tool – Chapter 9 Evolve
www.Smart2Smarter.com

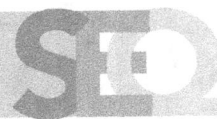
For academic course or corporate adoption and speaking engagements, contact Cynthia Kivland:
Cynthia@Smart2Smarter.com

Design by David Penna and Shawn Sargent
 www.davidpennastudios.com / www.shawnsargent.com

Copy editing and creative editing by Shawn Sargent
Layout and production by Shawn Sargent

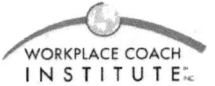

Smart2Smarter by Kivland, 2011 (www.smart2smarter.com)
For exclusive one time use by the Smart2Smarter Community and participants
in Social and Emotional Intelligence Coach or Leader Certification Program.
Workplace Coach Institute. © 2003-2010 Cynthia Kivland, President.
For group distribution or reproduction costs, contact cynthia@Smart2smarter.com

Chapter Nine - Evolve
Resource Tool

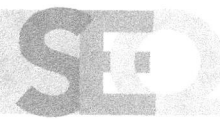
TABLE OF CONTENTS

Contents	Page
Career Health Inventory: Six Clusters	1
Organizational Health Inventory	1
Directions and Inventory	2-4
Scoring Your Results	5-6
Development Advice	7
Development Action Guide	8-18
Awareness Cluster	8-10
Strengths Cluster	10-11
Trends Cluster	12-13
Evolution Cluster	13-15
Reciprocity Cluster	15-16
Culture Cluster	17-18
SMARTER Reflections (blank page for notes)	19
Join the *Smart2Smarter* Career Community	20

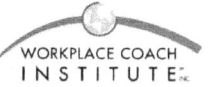

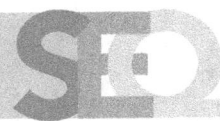
Join the Smart2Smarter Community
to *LIVE and WORK SMARTER*

smart *2* SMARTER
www.Smart2Smarter.com

smart 2 SMARTER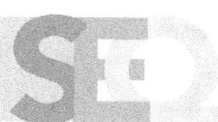

CAREER HEALTH INVENTORY AND DEVELOPMENT GUIDE

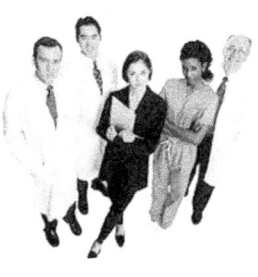

Maintaining your career health is similar to maintaining your physical health. Much like the regular preparation and conditioning athletes use to achieve in their sport, career health includes regular conditioning, practice and learning to evolve and achieve performance, career and lifestyle goals. A healthy career lifestyle establishes behavior habits and a mindset of continuous evolution that requires the intelligent use of your emotional, physical and social self. This tool provides a career health check-up, along with development activities to further condition your strengths and develop latent career health muscles.

The Career Health Inventory provides a snapshot in time by answering the following questions in six career health clusters:

Awareness Can you describe the core Career Management competencies to sustain your employability?

Strengths Can you describe your work skills, values, personality style and motivators that bring out your personal best?

Trends Can you describe the trends that are, and will, affect your industry and profession?

Evolve Do you have an evolution plan that includes continuous learning and skill development?

Reciprocity Do you regularly receive and give others information to help you and them to evolve?

Culture Are you working in a work environment that encourages and rewards career evolution?

Organizational Career Health

This inventory can provide a snapshot of your organization's career health by identifying the pressing career and coaching needs of your employees by demographics. The information will help your organization design and implement career and performance programs aligned with business goals. The inventory will be distributed in six to twelve months to assess progress towards developing individual and organization career fitness habits. Please contact Cynthia@Smart2Smarter.com or 1-877-60-COACH for more information.

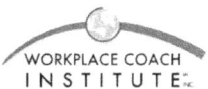

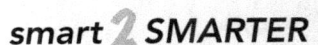
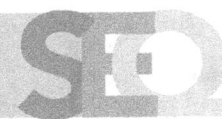
 ## CAREER HEALTH INVENTORY – SIX CLUSTERS

Directions

- Rate each of the following items by selecting the response that describes you or your work environment at this time.
- **Choose (5) if the statement describes you or your situation exactly, and (1) if the statement does not at all describe you or your situation.**
- This inventory takes five to seven minutes to complete.

	Cluster One: Career Awareness					
1.	I can state the difference between a job and a career.	1	2	3	4	5
2.	I can state the difference and link between performance and career development.	1	2	3	4	5
3.	I can state the six core Career Management competencies.	1	2	3	4	5
4.	I have used a formal process of career development in my work or academic life.	1	2	3	4	5
5.	I am aware of the process and purpose of my organization's career development system.	1	2	3	4	5
6.	I can clearly state my career goals for the next three years.	1	2	3	4	5
	Total Career Awareness					
	Cluster Two: Strengths					
7.	I know what skills I am good at and where I need to develop.	1	2	3	4	5
8.	I know my core values and how these guide my career decisions.	1	2	3	4	5
9.	I know what keeps me motivated to do my best work.	1	2	3	4	5
10.	I understand my basic personality and how this impacts my career evolution.	1	2	3	4	5
11.	I know the environment or culture that brings out my personal best.	1	2	3	4	5
12.	I have a written summary or portfolio of my career and life achievements.	1	2	3	4	5
	Total Strengths					

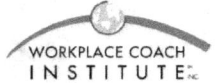 WORKPLACE COACH INSTITUTE

Smart2Smarter by Kivland, 2011 (www.smart2smarter.com)
For exclusive one time use by the Smart2Smarter Community and participants
in Social and Emotional Intelligence Coach or Leader Certification Program.
Workplace Coach Institute. © 2003-2010 Cynthia Kivland, President.
For group distribution or reproduction costs, contact cynthia@Smart2Smarter.com

Chapter Nine - Evolve
Resource Tool

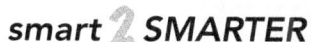
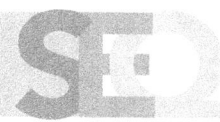
 ## CAREER HEALTH INVENTORY – SIX CLUSTERS

	Cluster Three: Trends – Industry/Political/Social/Economic					
13.	I know about industry and professional trends that may affect my employability.	1	2	3	4	5
14.	I regularly participate in development activities related to my profession, job or industry.	1	2	3	4	5
15.	I know where to find career and knowledge resources related to my profession or industry.	1	2	3	4	5
16.	I know the work competencies required of similar or advanced positions within my profession and industry.	1	2	3	4	5
17.	I know about general economic and societal trends that affect my industry or profession.	1	2	3	4	5
18.	I belong to a professional association or have professional colleagues to keep current on industry trends.	1	2	3	4	5
	Total Trends					
	Cluster Four: Evolve					
19.	I actively seek out work/school projects, classes or activities to apply new skills or to apply skills that stretch me beyond my comfort zones.	1	2	3	4	5
20.	I have identified performance areas where I need skill improvement.	1	2	3	4	5
21.	Each month, I participate in activities related to my career development plan on the job or outside of work.	1	2	3	4	5
22.	I have written career and performance goals, and have identified next steps to achieve these goals.	1	2	3	4	5
23.	Besides my manager, I know who in the organization has formal or informal influence to help me evolve.	1	2	3	4	5
24.	I know what internal and external development resources are available to achieve performance or career goals.	1	2	3	4	5
	Total Evolve					

CAREER HEALTH INVENTORY – SIX CLUSTERS

	Cluster Five: Reciprocity					
25.	I have recently initiated a conversation from a coworker about my performance.	1	2	3	4	5
26.	I have recently asked for a performance check-up from my manager outside of the formal review process.	1	2	3	4	5
27.	I have a work, community, professional or school-related network where I can give and receive to continually evolve.	1	2	3	4	5
28.	I have recently assisted a coworker with their development by listening and providing guidance.	1	2	3	4	5
29.	I have engaged in a career check-up from someone outside of my organization or profession (such as a career counselor or other helping professional).	1	2	3	4	5
30.	I have a performance or career discussion with my manager, coach or mentor at least once a month.	1	2	3	4	5
	Total Reciprocity					
	Cluster Six: Evolution Culture					
31.	My manager/college advisor feels comfortable discussing and supporting my career goals.	1	2	3	4	5
32.	My organization/school has a career development system in place to assist me with my career goals.	1	2	3	4	5
33.	My organization/school provides me with more than one annual performance or academic review.	1	2	3	4	5
34.	My organization/school rewards individuals who develop their work skills or assist others in skill development.	1	2	3	4	5
35.	My organization's/school's career development philosophy makes it an employer/school of choice, and I would refer people to this company/school.	1	2	3	4	5
36.	My organization/school has mentors or coaches to support my performance and career goals.	1	2	3	4	5
	Total Evolution Culture					

Smart2Smarter by Kivland, 2011 (www.smart2smarter.com)
For exclusive one time use by the Smart2Smarter Community and participants
in Social and Emotional Intelligence Coach or Leader Certification Program,
Workplace Coach Institute, © 2003-2010 Cynthia Kivland, President.
For group distribution or reproduction costs, contact cynthia@Smart2Smarter.com

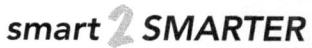 *smart* **2 SMARTER**

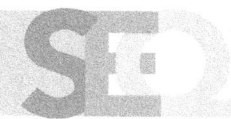

 CAREER HEALTH INVENTORY – SIX CLUSTERS SCORES AND RESULTS

Total Score Record your individual cluster score under the respective heading below. Then, add the six scores for a total Career Health score.

Awareness   _____
Strengths   _____
Trends   _____
Evolve   _____
Reciprocity   _____
Culture   _____
Total   _____

Your Individual Results

Awareness Awareness of the five Career Management competencies to sustain employability.
Strengths Knowledge of skills, values, personality and motivators that inspire your personal best.
Trends Trends that are, and will, affect your industry and profession.
Evolve Conditioning and practice plan that increases career success and significance.
Reciprocity Receive and give others feedback about work performance and career goals.
Culture Work/school environment encourages, inspires and rewards career evolution.

Step One

Your overall score provides a snapshot of your career health as measured by the six health clusters.

Total Score
144-180
You demonstrate consistent and focused career health habits. How do you reward yourself to sustain forward momentum? How can you be a coach to others on career fitness? What resources, people or shortcuts would you recommend to others that will help them evolve?

120-143
You sometimes practice career health habits to evolve and to sustain your employability. What stalls or disrupts your career fitness goals? Who can be part of your career health plan as an accountability partner? Focus first on fitness habits you do well, and strengthen them. Then choose one new habit to sharpen each month. It might be time to hire a coach to get you back on a regular and focused schedule to career health.

Less than 120
Time to develop career fitness habits to evolve to increase your employability, career success and significance. Choose accountability partner(s) to get you started and to keep you on your conditioning schedule. It might be time to hire a career coach!

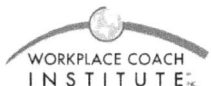

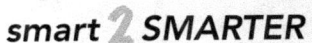 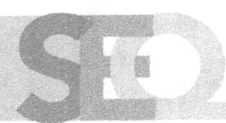
 MY CAREER HEALTH CLUSTER RESULTS

Step Two

Your cluster scores provide a snapshot of your established career health habits and those health habits that need improvement. Refer back to your career cluster scores and record below.

Consult the Career Health Development Activities chart to design a career fitness plan.

Awareness _____	Strengths _____	Trends _____
Evolve _____	Reciprocity _____	Culture _____	**Total** _____

My highest career cluster is _____.

This is an area that indicated strong career fitness habits.
Talk with your manager, college counselor, career coach or human resources representative to learn how you can share, showcase or further strengthen this career fitness habit.

The five highest statements that I rated *strongly agrees* with me are:

What is the common theme about the statements that you rated highest?

In what Career Health cluster(s) are these statements located?

What development activities are available internally and externally?

My lowest career cluster is _____.

This is an area for immediate emotional, skill or behavioral improvement.
Talk with your manager, college advisor, career professional, or human resources representative to learn what internal or external resources are available to improve this fitness habit.

The five statements that I rated *does not describe* me are:

What is the common theme related to the statements that you rated lowest?

In what Career Health cluster(s) are these statements located?

What development activities are available internally and externally?

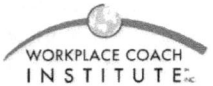

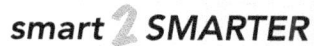 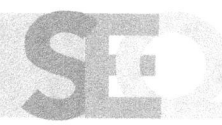
 ## CAREER HEALTH DEVELOPMENT ACTIVITIES

First, some development advice

Think about your development as an investment in your career satisfaction and performance success. A variety of development activities will give you a return on your investment. Remember, there are many paths to develop your career. Below are a few suggested actions to help focus your development commitment plan.

- **Modeling** Model individuals whose skills or workstyle you admire, or job tasks you want to perform.
- **Ask for Feedback** Strength of emotional intelligence is to ask for career guidance, performance feedback or professional advice regularly.
- **Find a Coach or Mentor** Coaches or mentors can advise how to develop and improve your skills, as well as keep you committed to a practice plan.
- **Classroom Training** Seek courses if you learn best in a classroom environment.
- **Practice Scrimmages** Athletes often have scrimmages; seek opportunities and projects to practice skill development.
- **Go Virtual** Use the Internet to search for distance learning classes, books and other resources to develop your career.
- **Create a Knowledge Network** Seek opportunities to exchange knowledge specific to your career or industry—whether in person or virtually.
- **Social Networking** Join social networks that align with your career interests.

Use the information from the Career Health Development Activities chart on the next several pages, along with feedback from your support team, to develop or enhance your career health.

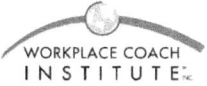

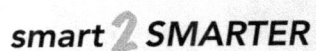 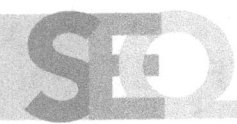

 CAREER HEALTH DEVELOPMENT ACTIVITIES

Competency Cluster	Appraisal Factor	Forward Action Development Activities
Career Awareness	Know the difference between a job and a career.	Commit to learn these definitions! **Job** Arbitrary way to package work and projects that need to be done to achieve business or organizational goals. Jobs are composed of specific tasks and competencies in a given profession. **Career** The work roles you perform over the course of your lifetime, often related to a profession. **Profession** A recognized area of expertise and discipline that is enduring and has recognized leaders, educational programs, professional associations and publications.
Career Awareness	Know the difference between performance and career development.	Know your organization's or school's definition of performance and career development. **Performance Management** Focuses on a twelve-month plan to develop knowledge and competencies important to current or future business goals. You and your manager jointly own the development plan driven by business, department or job function goals identified during the review or appraisal process. **Career Development** A continuous process that encompasses both work and lifestyle goals. Your career development plan usually extends one to three years, with adjustment of goals and focus in relation to life/work changes. It is owned and guided by an individual's interests, values, life circumstances or skills rather than the tactical needs of annual performance goals.

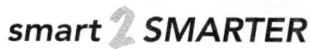

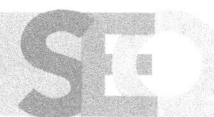

 CAREER HEALTH DEVELOPMENT ACTIVITIES ────────────────

Competency Cluster	Appraisal Factor	Forward Action Development Activities
Career Awareness	Know the five Career Resilient Success Factors recognized by the *National Association of Career Management Professionals*. You can visit www.ncda.org.	Learn the five Career Resilient Success Factors. Take the Career Resilience Inventory available in the book *Smart 2 Smarter.* **Self-Knowledge** Skills to regularly gather self-knowledge about work/life needs and goals. **Career Transition** Skills and resources to manage life and career transitions. **Career Information** Skills to locate, evaluate and interpret career information. **Career Search** Skills to obtain, maintain or change one's career or job position. **Self-Promotion** Skills that actively promote and market oneself within or outside the organization to align one's natural career passion with performance and business results. **Ask** What Success Factor needs immediate development?
Career Awareness	Usage of career development services in your academic or work life.	What stopped or stalled you from using the services in the past? What benefit did you receive from using these services? Research organizational, community, library, school or Internet resources that are available to develop your career. Commit to visit three within the next four weeks.

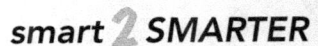 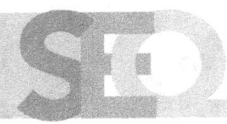
 CAREER HEALTH DEVELOPMENT ACTIVITIES

Competency Cluster	Appraisal Factor	Forward Action Development Activities
Career Awareness	Knowledge of your organization's or school's career development resources.	Ask your human resources representative, coach, manager or college advisor to describe the programs and resources available for career development. Commit to research three resources or programs within the next four weeks.
Career Awareness	Written statement of career goals for the next three years.	Ask your manager, coach, human resources representative or college advisor about resources available to write a career plan including a goal planning worksheet. Commit to draft a written career plan during the next four weeks.
Strengths	Knowledge of the skills which you do well and the skills you can teach to others.	Ask others what skills they see you as doing well or that you can teach to others. Ask your human resources representative, manager, coach or college advisor to describe the resources or assessments available to gain a realistic appraisal of your values. Construct a list of achievements in your work, personal, community or leisure life and list the skills you used. Schedule a meeting with your manager to get feedback on your skill assessment. Take a skill assessment that measures both job function and interpersonal skills during the next four weeks.

WORKPLACE COACH
I N S T I T U T E

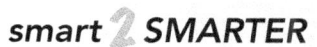
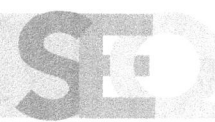
 ## CAREER HEALTH DEVELOPMENT ACTIVITIES

Competency Cluster	Appraisal Factor	Forward Action Development Activities
Strengths	Knowledge of the core values that guide your career decisions.	Ask your human resources representative, manager, coach or college advisor to describe the resources or assessments available to gain a realistic appraisal of your values. Commit to take a Values Assessment within the next four weeks.
Strengths	Knowledge of work environment motivators that influence you to perform at your best.	Ask your human resources representative, manager or college advisor to describe the resources or assessments available to gain a realistic appraisal of your work environment and career interest motivators. Commit to take a Work Environment or Interest Assessment within the next four weeks.
Strengths	Knowledge of your personality style and how it influences my career satisfaction.	Ask your human resources representative, coach, manager or college advisor to describe the resources or assessments available to gain a realistic appraisal of your personality style. Commit to take a Personality Style Assessment within the next four weeks.
Strengths	Written summary or portfolio of my career/life achievements.	Ask your human resources representative, coach, manager or college advisor to describe the resources available to draft a written summary of your career/life achievements. Gather documents and work/school products that summarize key career achievements. Create a folder or purchase a binder to record and store your career/life achievements. Update your resume and online profile to reflect your latest achievements every three months.

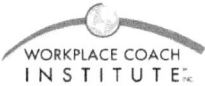

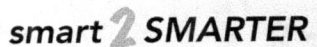 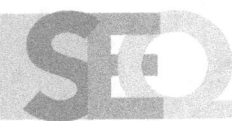

 ## CAREER HEALTH DEVELOPMENT ACTIVITIES

Competency Cluster	Appraisal Factor	Forward Action Development Activities
Trends	I know where to find information about industry and professional trends that affect my employability.	Ask your human resources representative, coach, manager or college advisor to describe where to locate resources about employment trends. Commit to locate four resources within the next four weeks.
Trends	I participate in development activities related to my profession or job.	Ask your human resources representative, coach, manager or college advisor to describe development activities specific to your job or career available within or outside the company. Commit to research four development activities or internal training programs. Choose to participate or register for one activity in the next four weeks.
Trends	I belong to a professional association related to my profession or industry.	Ask your human resources representative, coach, peer, manager or college advisor about professional associations related to your profession or industry. Commit to join one professional association or social networking group within the next two months. Commit to an active role in the association as part of your career plan.
Trends	I know the emerging work competencies of similar or advanced positions within my profession and industry.	Ask your human resources representative, coach, peer, manager or college advisor about emerging work competencies of similar or advanced positions within your industry or profession. Interview a colleague or peer who has a position that you aspire to achieve. Ask what skills/competencies are important to obtain and be successful in that position. Attend professional conferences or association meetings to learn what skills or knowledge employers want in your job function or career path.

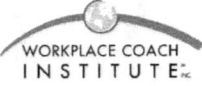

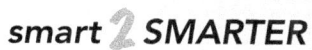
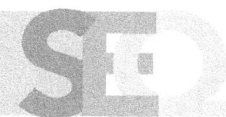
 ## CAREER HEALTH DEVELOPMENT ACTIVITIES

Competency Cluster	Appraisal Factor	Forward Action Development Activities
Trends	I know about general economic and societal trends that may affect my industry or profession.	Ask your human resources representative, coach, manager or college advisor about industry or professional resources to stay current on trends. Ask your manager about trends or events outside of your department or company. Subscribe and contribute to journals, blogs or social networking groups to stay current and connected. Attend and contribute to webinars, conferences or associations to learn about trends.
Trends	I meet regularly with professional colleagues to keep current on industry trends.	Select a Board of Directors of peers or mentors to keep current on industry trends. Commit to meet monthly by phone or in person to keep your career on track with industry trends. Schedule a meeting date to confer with a peer(s) or mentor within the next four weeks.
Evolution Plan	I actively seek work projects to apply new skills or those that require the learning of new skills.	Ask your human resources representative, coach, peer, manager or college advisor about emerging work skills of similar or advanced positions within your industry or profession. Include a goal on your performance or career plan to commit to one new project or activity that requires new skills or knowledge. Seek community or association events that require you to apply new learning or skills.

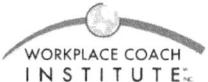

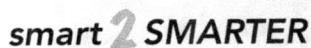 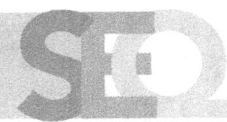
 CAREER HEALTH DEVELOPMENT ACTIVITIES

Competency Cluster	Appraisal Factor	Forward Action Development Activities
Evolution Plan	I have identified and discussed with my manager the performance areas where I need skill improvement.	Meet with your manager to identify performance areas that you mutually agree need improvement. Ask your manager for a career health check-up that will identify target areas for improvement. Agree with your manager on up to five areas for immediate improvement that directly relate to job, department, team or business goals.
Evolution Plan	Each month, I participate in activities related to my career development plan on the job or outside of work.	Write in your development plan specific monthly activities to evolve and sustain your employability. Ask to meet monthly with your manager, coach, peer or college advisor for review and support. Reward yourself for attending development events. Keep a written record in your portfolio of the events you attended and development outcomes.
Evolution Plan	I have written career and performance goals, and have next steps to achieve these goals.	Ask your human resources representative, coach, peer, manager or college advisor about resources, worksheets or forms to assist you in preparing written career and performance goals. Use the SMARTER method of goal setting. Attend a goal-setting seminar or read a book about goal setting.
Evolution Plan	Besides my manager, I know who in the organization or school has accountability to assist with my performance and career goals.	Ask your human resources representative, advisor, manager or peer about who can assist with your career development. Meet with that person within four weeks to learn how this person will be an asset to your career or performance goals and plans.

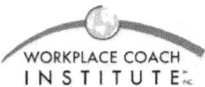

Smart2Smarter by Kiviand, 2011 (www.smart2smarter.com)
For exclusive one time use by the Smart2Smarter Community and participants
in Social and Emotional Intelligence Coach or Leader Certification Program.
Workplace Coach Institute. © 2003-2010 Cynthia Kiviand, President.
For group distribution or reproduction costs, contact cynthia@Smart2Smarter.com

Chapter Nine - Evolve
Resource Tool

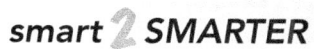
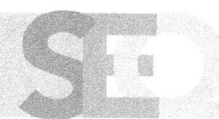
 ## CAREER HEALTH DEVELOPMENT ACTIVITIES

Competency Cluster	Appraisal Factor	Forward Action Development Activities
Evolution Plan	I know what internal and external development resources are available to increase my career satisfaction or performance success.	Ask your human resources representative, manager, coach, college advisor or peers what resources are available inside of the organization and what community or distance learning resources are recommended that can assist with your career or performance development. Make a commitment to research three of these resources within the next four weeks. Choose one activity for your evolution plan.
Reciprocity	I have recently asked for feedback on my performance from a co-worker.	Seek out a co-worker and ask for performance feedback about a specific project or job task. Ask your human resources department about peer reviews or 360° Feedback process. Commit to a monthly feedback check-up with a co-worker, and schedule a regular date.
Reciprocity	I have recently asked for feedback on performance from my manager outside of the formal review process.	Schedule a meeting with your manager to discuss your performance or development goals at least every two months. Ask human resources, your coach or manager for performance discussion worksheets or forms that will facilitate the process. Prepare an updated list of accomplishments and outcomes for the development discussion. Bring documents, work product and/or testimonials.

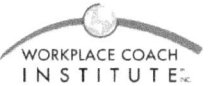

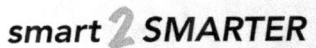
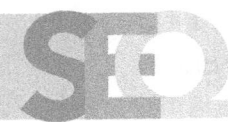
 CAREER HEALTH DEVELOPMENT ACTIVITIES

Competency Cluster	Appraisal Factor	Forward Action Development Activities
Reciprocity	I have a work-related professional network where I can give and receive feedback.	Choose no more than five colleagues to serve as your personal Board of Directors or accountability partners. Meet with colleagues monthly, by phone, in person or via social networks to give and receive feedback about your career. Schedule a first meeting within the next four weeks.
Reciprocity	I have recently assisted a coworker with their career development by giving them constructive feedback.	Ask your manager for opportunities to be a mentor to co-workers. Collaborate with a co-worker to arrange a monthly peer-shared review career check-up. Seek programs or development activities to develop mentoring skills.
Reciprocity	I have asked for career feedback from someone outside of my organization or profession (such as a career coach or other helping professional).	Research career professionals recommended by your company, college, peer or community resources. Set an informational meeting to learn how she or he assists individuals with career and performance goals. Check references and credentials.
Reciprocity	I have a performance or career discussion with my manager, coach or mentor at least once a month.	Schedule "Focus on Me" development dates in your monthly planner. Vary the feedback mechanism and the person, whether in person or by phone. Schedule a monthly career fitness date and identify the person within the next four weeks. Confirm the date and the focus of the development discussion with that individual.

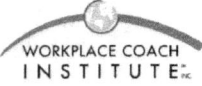

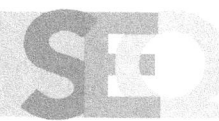
 CAREER HEALTH DEVELOPMENT ACTIVITIES

Competency Cluster	Appraisal Factor	Forward Action Development Activities
Culture	My manager has the skills to discuss and support my career goals.	Ask your human resources representative or peers about management/leadership training on conducting career discussions. Recommend skill training for staff and managers on how to conduct and prepare for development discussions. Research coaches, courses, books or resources to upgrade manager's coaching skills.
Culture	My organization has a career development system to assist me with my career goals.	Ask your manager what resources are available to assist with your development, both career and performance. Meet with human resources staff to learn about development programs and services. Volunteer to benchmark what organizations in your industry or profession are offering to retain and develop talent. Contact a career coach or consultant to conduct a career systems audit.
Culture	My organization has internal or external mentors or coaches to facilitate my performance and career goals.	Ask your manager about coaches or mentors that can assist with your development, both career and performance. Meet with human resources staff to learn about mentoring programs or coaching services.
Culture	My organization rewards individuals who develop their skills or assist others in skill development.	Ask your manager about reward systems aligned with obtaining performance or development goals. Ask your manager about rewards systems aligned with teaching or mentoring others. If you have direct reports, construct and communicate reward systems for obtaining development/performance goals *or* assisting others in obtainment of their goals.

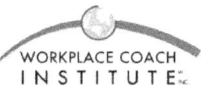

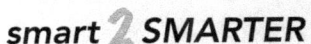
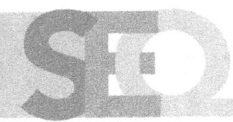
 ## CAREER HEALTH DEVELOPMENT ACTIVITIES

Competency Cluster	Appraisal Factor	Forward Action Development Activities
Culture	My organization's career development philosophy makes it an employer of choice, and I would refer people to work for this company.	Does your organization have a referral policy? If so, how many recent hires were referred by existing employees. If you are a manager, do you know why your star performers stay or leave? Gather information from colleagues, professional associations or Internet sites about the talent development practices of similar industries or companies.

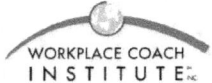 WORKPLACE COACH INSTITUTE

Chapter Nine - Evolve
Resource Tool

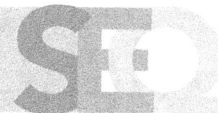
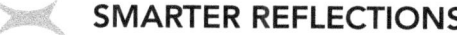

SMARTER REFLECTIONS

Use this space to record your thoughts and reflections about the information in this resource

Join the SMARTER Community To Bring Humanity and Civility Back Into the Workplace!

What will you find on Smart2Smarter.com?

- Over 100 social and emotional intelligence tools

- Daily skill-building workouts

- Downloadable coaching activities and articles

- SMARTER career nuggets for smart people and leaders

- Workplace training and coach certification programs on leadership, resilience, career direction, emotional intelligence, empathy and more

- Seamless online ordering

- Guidelines and information on how to become a *Smart2Smarter* affiliate

- Global community of authors, researchers, consultants and coaches

This is the first website dedicated to bringing humanity and civility back into the workplace...

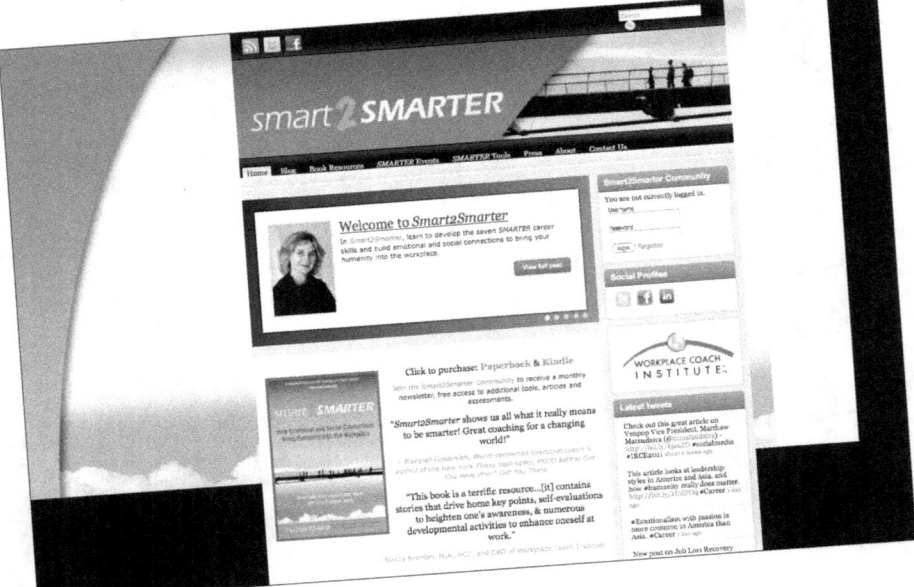

To inquire about having Cynthia speak at your next conference, workplace or special event, contact: Cynthia@Smart2Smarter.com

www.ingramcontent.com/pod-product-compliance
Lightning Source LLC
Chambersburg PA
CBHW081812280526
45789CB00008B/3110